28-DAYS WALL PILATES CHALLENGE FOR WOMEN OVER 50

EASY STEP BY STEP GUIDE FOR YOU TO LOSE WEIGHT, IMPROVE BALANCE, MOBILITY, FLEXIBILITY AND STRENGTH THROUGH THIS PILATES EXERCISES.

Ronald Mullins

TABLE OF CONTENT

INTRODUCTION 7

CHAPTER 1 11

Understanding Wall Pilates for Women Over 50 11

Why Wall Pilates 13

Benefits of Wall Pilates 16

CHAPTER 2 19

Preparing Your Space and Equipment......................................19

Safety Tips and Precautions..21

How to Use This Book Effectively 24

CHAPTER 3 27

Week 1: Posture and Alignment Awareness................................27

Goals for Week 1:..27

Benefits for Week 1:...27

Day 1: Welcome to the Pilates Challenge..................................28

Day 2: Posture and Alignment Techniques.................................30

Day 3: Activating the Deep Core Muscles..................................31

Day 4: Breathing Techniques for Mind-Body Connection 33

Day 5: Developing Pelvic Floor Strength 34

Day 6: Balance and Stability Exercises 36

Day 7: Weekly Progress Check and Reflection 37

CHAPTER 4 39

Week 2: Mobility and Flexibility Enhancement 39

Goals for Week 2: 39

Benefits for Week 2: 39

Day 8: Increasing Spinal Flexibility 41

Day 9: Shoulder Mobility and Strength 42

Day 10: Hip Flexibility and Range of Motion 44

Day 11: Unlocking Hamstring and Hip Flexor Tightness.............45

Day 12: Enhancing Joint Mobility Safely.....................................46

Day 13: Pilates Stretches for Whole-Body Flexibility..................48

Day 14: Weekly Progress Check and Reflection 49

CHAPTER 5 51

Week 3: Strength and Muscle Tone Development 51

Goals for week 3: 51

Benefits for week 3: 51

Day 15: Introduction to Pilates Resistance Training......................52

Day 16: Building Upper Body Strength...........................54

Day 17: Lower Body Muscle Activation 55

Day 18: Core Strengthening Progressions 56

Day 19: Full-Body Resistance Exercises 57

Day 20: Incorporating Small Equipment for Added Challenge 58

Day 21: Weekly Progress Check and Reflection 60

CHAPTER 6...62

Week 4: Balance and Coordination Enhancement....................62

Goals for week 4:...62

Benefits for week 4:..62

Day 22: Understanding Balance and Coordination................64

Day 23: Basic Balance Exercises.................................65

Day 24: Advanced Balance and Core Integration.................66

Day 25: Dynamic Balance and Coordination Challenges...........67

Day 26: Integrating Balance and Strength 69

Day 27: Balance and Coordination Flow 70

Day 28: Final Progress Check and Reflection 70

Conclusion..73

INTRODUCTION

Welcome to the 28 Days Wall Pilates Challenge for Women Over 50! This book is designed to be your companion on a transformative journey towards improved fitness, strength, flexibility, and overall well-being. If you're a woman over 50 who's looking to enhance your physical health, boost your energy levels, and experience the joy of movement, you're in the right place.

Pilates is a fantastic exercise method that offers numerous benefits, especially for individuals in the 50+ age group. It focuses on building core strength, improving posture, increasing flexibility, and fostering a mind-body connection that contributes to better balance and overall functionality. In this challenge, you'll discover how Pilates, combined with the support of a wall for added stability, can become a powerful tool for achieving your fitness goals and embracing a healthier lifestyle.

This book is not just about exercise; it's about empowerment. It's about dedicating 28 days to yourself, acknowledging the importance of self-care, and embarking on a journey that celebrates your body's capabilities and your own inner strength. Each day's practice will bring you closer to your goals, and by the end of this challenge, you'll not only feel physically transformed but also mentally rejuvenated.

Karen, a vibrant woman in her early 50s, was feeling the weight of age gradually creeping into her daily life. She longed for a way to regain her vitality and embrace the years ahead with renewed strength. One day, while browsing online, she stumbled upon the "28 Days Wall Pilates Challenge for Women Over 50." Intrigued, she decided to embark on this journey.

During the first week, Karen discovered the power of posture. As she engaged her core and aligned her body, she felt an immediate lightness and reduction in back discomfort. Breathing techniques became her sanctuary, helping her stay calm amidst life's chaos.

In the second week, flexibility was her focus. Karen marveled at her newfound ability to touch her toes without strain. Her hips felt more fluid, and her once-tight shoulders began to relax. Each stretch became a reminder of her body's incredible resilience.

As she entered the strength-focused third week, Karen surprised herself. Lifting weights and performing resistance exercises made her feel strong and empowered. Her posture improved even further, and her walks felt effortless.

In the final week, balance and coordination became her allies. Karen noticed herself walking with newfound grace, navigating challenges with poise. She marveled at her body's ability to adapt.

As the challenge concluded, Karen reflected on her transformation. The challenge wasn't just about physical changes; it was about embracing her body's potential. She now faced life with a vibrant spirit, empowered by the lessons learned over 28 days. The challenge had not only revitalized her body but also reignited her zest for life.

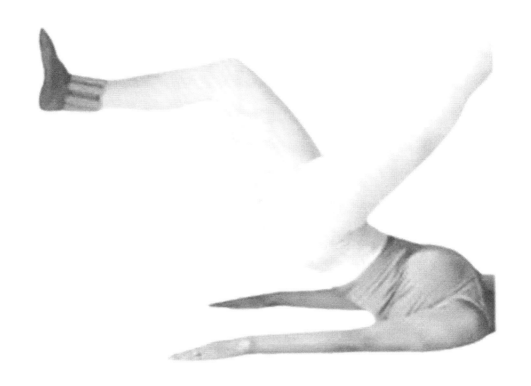

CHAPTER 1

Understanding Wall Pilates for Women Over 50

In this chapter, we delve into the heart of the 28 Days Wall Pilates Challenge, focusing on understanding the practice of Wall Pilates specifically tailored for women over 50. This section will provide you with comprehensive insights into the unique benefits, principles, and techniques that make Wall Pilates an ideal exercise method for your age group.

Benefits of Wall Pilates for Women Over 50:

Discover the multitude of advantages that Wall Pilates offers specifically to women over 50. From core strengthening to improving flexibility, posture, and balance, this section will highlight how Wall Pilates addresses the specific needs and challenges that often arise as women enter this stage of life. Gain a clear understanding of how Wall Pilates can support your overall well-being and enhance your quality of life.

Mind-Body Connection and Wall Pilates:

One of the distinguishing features of Wall Pilates is its emphasis on the mind-body connection. Learn how this practice encourages mindfulness and awareness during movement, fostering a deeper connection to your body. By cultivating this connection, you can enhance your exercise experience, reduce stress, and promote a positive outlook on your fitness journey.

Adapting Wall Pilates to Your Needs:

Every individual's body is unique, and as a woman over 50, you may have specific considerations and goals. This section will guide you on how to adapt Wall Pilates exercises to your personal needs and abilities. Whether you're a beginner or have experience with Pilates, these insights will empower you to tailor your practice for optimal results and comfort.

Mindful Movement and Breathing Techniques:

Central to Wall Pilates is the integration of breath and movement. Learn how mindful breathing techniques enhance the effectiveness of each exercise and promote relaxation. By aligning your breath with your movements, you'll cultivate a sense of presence and harmony that contributes to both your physical and mental well-being.

Why Wall Pilates

As women progress into their 50s and beyond, maintaining their physical health and well-being becomes increasingly vital. This life stage often brings about various changes in the body, such as decreased bone density, muscle mass, and flexibility. This is why incorporating a fitness routine tailored to the unique needs of women over 50 is essential. Wall Pilates emerges as a highly effective and relevant exercise method for this demographic. Here's why:

1. Safe and Supportive: Wall Pilates provides a stable surface for exercise, ensuring safety and reducing the risk of injury. For women over 50 who may be more prone to joint sensitivities or balance issues, having the wall as support can instill confidence and allow for a controlled range of motion.

2. Core Focus for Posture and Stability: As the body ages, maintaining good posture becomes crucial to prevent discomfort and support spinal health. Wall Pilates places a strong emphasis on core strengthening, which contributes to improved posture and stability. Strengthening the core muscles helps women over 50 stand tall, move with grace, and reduce the strain on the back and neck.

3. Bone Health and Strength: One of the key concerns for women in this age group is maintaining bone health and preventing osteoporosis. Wall Pilates incorporates weight-bearing exercises that stimulate bone growth, helping to enhance bone density and minimize the risk of fractures.

4. Gentle Joint Movement: Wall Pilates exercises are designed to be gentle on the joints while still promoting mobility. The controlled and mindful movements help to maintain joint flexibility and prevent stiffness that often comes with age.

5. Mindfulness and Stress Reduction: Women over 50 often encounter increased stress due to life changes and responsibilities. Wall Pilates integrates mindfulness and controlled breathing techniques, which not only enhance the effectiveness of the exercises but also promote relaxation and stress reduction.

6. Balance and Fall Prevention: Maintaining balance and preventing falls become essential as we age. Wall Pilates incorporates exercises that challenge balance and coordination, contributing to improved stability and reduced risk of accidents.

7. Confidence and Empowerment: Engaging in regular physical activity, such as Wall Pilates, instills a sense of accomplishment and empowerment. Women over 50 can experience an increased sense of confidence in their bodies and capabilities, which positively impacts their overall well-being.

8. Holistic Well-Being: Wall Pilates isn't just about physical exercise; it's a holistic approach that connects the body and mind. This comprehensive practice can improve mood, boost energy levels, and promote a greater sense of well-being.

9. Adaptability to Fitness Levels: Whether you're new to exercise or have been active throughout your life, Wall Pilates is adaptable to various fitness levels. The use of the wall as support allows individuals to progress at their own pace and gradually challenge themselves.

10. Lifelong Wellness: The benefits of Wall Pilates extend far beyond the challenge's duration. By embracing Wall Pilates as part of a regular fitness routine, women over 50 can enjoy improved health, vitality, and quality of life well into their later years.

Incorporating Wall Pilates into your fitness journey can be a transformative experience that addresses the specific needs of women over 50.

Benefits of Wall Pilates

Pilates is a holistic exercise method that offers a multitude of advantages, especially for women over 50. As your body experiences natural changes with age, incorporating Pilates into your fitness routine can provide remarkable benefits that contribute to your overall well-being. You might anticipate to gain from the following main advantages:

1. Core Strength: wall Pilates focuses on building core strength, which is essential for stability, balance, and supporting your spine. Strengthening your core can help alleviate back pain and improve your posture, allowing you to stand tall and move with greater ease.

2. Flexibility: wall Pilates exercises emphasize elongating muscles and increasing flexibility. Improved flexibility can enhance your range of motion, making everyday activities more comfortable and reducing the risk of injury.

3. Posture Improvement: The mind-body connection inherent in Pilates encourages awareness of your body's alignment. By practicing proper posture during exercises, you'll carry this awareness into your daily life, reducing strain on your muscles and joints.

4. Bone Health: Weight-bearing exercises, common in Pilates, promote bone health and density. This is crucial for women over 50, as it can help reduce the risk of osteoporosis and fractures.

5. Joint Mobility: wall Pilates movements focus on fluidity and controlled motion, promoting joint mobility. This can ease joint stiffness and discomfort, allowing you to move more comfortably.

6. Muscle Tone: wall Pilates engages both large and small muscle groups, leading to improved muscle tone and a leaner appearance. Strengthening these muscles contributes to better metabolism and overall energy levels.

7. Mind-Body Connection: wall Pilates encourages mindfulness and concentration during exercises. This mental engagement not only improves the effectiveness of the workout but also helps you stay present and reduce stress.

8. Balance and Stability: wall Pilates exercises often challenge balance and stability, which are crucial skills for maintaining independence as you age. These exercises help prevent falls and enhance confidence in your movements.

9. Stress Reduction: The controlled breathing and mindfulness aspects of Pilates can promote relaxation and stress reduction. This is particularly beneficial for managing stress that can accompany the challenges of aging.

10. Joint-Friendly: wall Pilates is low-impact and gentle on the joints, making it suitable for women over 50 who may have joint sensitivities. It provides an effective workout without putting unnecessary strain on the body.

11. Overall Well-Being: The combination of physical exercise, mental focus, and mind-body connection in Pilates can lead to a greater sense of well-being and vitality, helping you embrace life's challenges with a positive outlook.

As you embark on the 28 Days Wall Pilates Challenge, keep these benefits in mind. With consistent practice and dedication, you'll experience the transformative power of Pilates and discover how it can enhance your physical health, mental clarity, and overall quality of life.

CHAPTER 2

Preparing Your Space and Equipment

Creating an optimal environment for your 28 Days Wall Pilates Challenge is essential to ensure a comfortable, focused, and safe practice. This chapter provides a comprehensive guide to setting up your practice space and gathering the necessary equipment. By dedicating time to these preparations, you'll create a supportive backdrop for your transformative journey.

Designing Your Practice Space:

Choose a space in your home that allows you to move freely and comfortably. Here's how to create an inviting and functional practice area:

1. Clear the Area: Remove any obstacles or clutter that could hinder your movement. Create ample space around you for the full range of exercises.

2. Lighting: opt for natural light, when possible, as it boosts your mood and enhances visibility. If natural light isn't available, ensure your practice area is well-lit to prevent strain.

3. Ventilation: Adequate airflow is crucial. Choose a space with good ventilation to keep you comfortable throughout your practice.

4. Distractions: Minimize distractions such as phones, computers, or noisy areas. Designate this space as a sanctuary for your practice.

Gathering Your Equipment

To fully engage in the Wall Pilates Challenge, gather the following items:

1. Wall Space: Find a clear section of wall that is sturdy and stable. This wall will be your support and guide throughout the challenge.

2. Mat: A supportive exercise mat provides cushioning for your body during exercises and ensures a comfortable practice.

4. Water Bottle and Towel: Stay hydrated and have a towel nearby to wipe off sweat.

5. Comfortable Attire: Wear comfortable, non-restrictive clothing that allows you to move freely. Choose breathable fabrics that facilitate movement.

Safety Tips and Precautions

Prioritizing your safety is paramount as you embark on the 28 Days Wall Pilates Challenge. This chapter provides a comprehensive guide to ensure you practice Wall Pilates in a safe and mindful manner. By following these safety tips and precautions, you'll reduce the risk of injury and create an environment that promotes your overall well-being.

1. Warm-Up and Cool Down:

Always begin your practice with a gentle warm-up to gradually elevate your heart rate and prepare your muscles for movement. Likewise, conclude your practice with a cool-down to help your body transition back to a resting state. These steps support flexibility and prevent strain.

2. Listen to Your Body:

During each exercise, pay special attention to how your body feels. If you experience pain, discomfort, or excessive strain, stop the exercise immediately. Remember that discomfort is different from challenge— never push yourself beyond your limits.

3. Proper Form and Alignment:

Maintaining proper form is crucial for effective and safe practice. Follow the instructions carefully for each exercise to ensure you're engaging the correct muscles and minimizing the risk of injury. Proper alignment helps distribute stress evenly through your body.

4. Breathing:

Breath awareness is integral to Wall Pilates. Breathe deeply and rhythmically, engaging your diaphragm. Sync your breath with your movements to facilitate controlled and focused exercises.

5. Avoid Overexertion:

While challenging yourself is essential, avoid overexertion. Gradually progress through exercises, and don't rush the process. Consistency and gradual improvement yield better results than pushing too hard.

6. Hydration and Nutrition:

Stay hydrated throughout your practice. Have a water bottle nearby and take sips as needed. Fuel your body with a balanced meal or snack before practicing to ensure you have the energy to engage effectively.

7. Avoid Sharp Movements:

Pilates emphasizes controlled and flowing movements. Avoid sudden or jerky motions that can strain muscles or joints. Smooth, controlled movements maximize the benefits of your practice.

8. Modify as Needed:

If an exercise is too challenging or causes discomfort, feel free to modify or skip it. Use props or variations to accommodate your body's needs and limitations.

9. Consult a Professional:

If you have any existing medical conditions or concerns, consult a healthcare professional before starting the challenge. Depending on your particular requirements, they can offer you individualized advice.

How to Use This Book Effectively

Congratulations on embarking on the 28 Days Wall Pilates Challenge for Women Over 50! To make the most of this book and ensure a successful and rewarding experience, here are some guidelines on how to use it effectively:

1. Understand the Structure: Familiarize yourself with the table of contents to understand the layout of the book. Each chapter corresponds to a week of the challenge, and each day within the chapters presents a new exercise or focus.

2. Read the Introduction: Begin by reading the introduction to gain a clear understanding of the purpose and benefits of the challenge. This will set the tone for your journey and motivate you to commit fully.

3. Gather Equipment: Take note of the equipment needed for the challenge, especially the use of a wall for support. Ensure you have a clear space to practice and any additional props required for specific exercises.

4. Set Realistic Goals: Before you start, set clear and achievable goals for yourself. These could be related to core strength, flexibility, posture improvement, or any other aspect you wish to focus on during the challenge.

5. Progress Gradually: The challenge is designed with a progressive structure, starting with foundational exercises and gradually advancing. Follow the sequence as outlined in the book to build a strong foundation and prevent injury.

6. Prioritize Consistency: Consistency is key to achieving results. Commit to practicing each day's exercises and stick to the recommended schedule. If you miss a day, don't worry—simply pick up where you left off and continue.

7. Listen to Your Body: Pay close attention to your body's signals. If an exercise feels too challenging or causes discomfort, modify it or skip it. The goal is to work within your comfort zone while gradually pushing your limits.

8. Focus on Form: Proper form is essential for effective and safe practice. Read the instructions carefully for each exercise and follow the cues provided to ensure you're performing them correctly.

9. Use the Review Days: Take advantage of the review days at the end of each week to reflect on your progress. Use this time to note any changes you've observed in your strength, flexibility, or overall well-being.

10. Document Your Journey: Consider keeping a journal to record your thoughts, observations, and any changes you experience throughout the challenge. This documentation can be a valuable way to track your progress and stay motivated.

CHAPTER 3

Week 1: Posture and Alignment Awareness

Understanding the Foundations of Good Posture

Goals for Week 1:

1. Develop an awareness of your current posture and alignment.

2. Understand the principles of proper posture and alignment.

3. Learn to engage your core muscles to support your posture.

4. Practice breath coordination to enhance your body's alignment.

5. Explore exercises that improve your pelvic floor strength.

6. Cultivate mindfulness and body awareness in daily activities.

Benefits for Week 1:

1. Improved Posture: Develop awareness of your posture and learn techniques to maintain proper alignment for reduced strain on your body.

2. Enhanced Core Strength: Engage your core muscles to support your spine, leading to improved stability and reduced risk of back pain.

3. Better Breathing: Practice breath coordination techniques that improve oxygenation, reduce tension, and enhance overall relaxation.

4. Pelvic Floor Health: Strengthen your pelvic floor muscles, which can contribute to improved bladder control and core stability.

5. Increased Body Awareness: Develop mindfulness and body awareness that positively influence your daily movements and habits.

Welcome to Week 1 of the 28 Days Wall Pilates Challenge for Women Over 50. This week is all about building a solid foundation and developing core awareness. These fundamental principles are essential for a successful and safe Pilates journey. We'll guide you through each day's activities, providing step-by-step instructions to ensure you get the most out of your practice.

Day 1: Welcome to the Pilates Challenge

Introduction to Pilates for Women Over 50

Overview:

Welcome to the 28-day Pilates challenge tailored specifically for women over 50. Pilates is a holistic approach to physical fitness that focuses on core strength, flexibility, and posture. This challenge is designed to help you experience the numerous benefits of Pilates, including improved strength, balance, and overall well-being.

Activity:

1. Find a Quiet Space: Choose a quiet and comfortable space where you can focus without distractions.

2. Wear Comfortable Clothing: Put on comfortable, breathable clothing that allows for free movement.

3. Warm-Up: Start with a brief warm-up. March in place or perform gentle shoulder rolls for 5 minutes to prepare your body for movement.

4. Breathing Exercise: Sit or stand comfortably. Close your eyes and take a deep breath in through your nose, expanding your ribcage. By using your mouth to exhale deeply, you can totally clear your lungs. By using your mouth to exhale deeply, you can totally clear your lungs, Repeat this for 5 cycles. This exercise helps you become aware of your breath, a crucial aspect of Pilates.

5. Gentle Stretches: Perform gentle stretches for your neck, shoulders, and back to release tension.

6. Mindful Intention: Set an intention for this challenge. What do you hope to achieve? Whether it's improved posture, increased strength, or reduced stress, make it a part of your journey.

Day 2: Posture and Alignment Techniques

Understanding the Importance of Posture in Pilates

Overview:

Proper posture is the foundation of Pilates. Good posture not only enhances your appearance but also plays a significant role in preventing discomfort and injury. In this session, you'll learn about alignment and how to maintain it during your Pilates practice.

Activity:

1. Body Scan: Stand with your feet hip-width apart. Do a quick body check while you are closed-eyed. Are you leaning forward, backward, or to the sides? Note any areas of tension or discomfort.

2. Neutral Spine: The neutral spine is the ideal alignment for Pilates. Imagine a straight line running through your head, shoulders, spine, and pelvis. Practice maintaining this alignment as you stand.

3. Wall Exercise: Stand with your back against a wall, heels about 4 inches away. Gently press your lower back, middle back, and upper back against the wall. Your head should be touching the wall as well. Hold this position for 30 seconds while focusing on your breath.

4. Pelvic Tilt: Stand away from the wall. Place your hands on your hips. Inhale to prepare, exhale, and gently tuck your pelvis under, as if you're trying to pull your belly button toward your spine. Inhale to release. Repeat this movement for 10 breath cycles.

5. Alignment Check: Stand in front of a mirror and assess your posture. Are you standing taller and with improved alignment? Make mental notes of how it feels to stand in a neutral spine position.

Day 3: Activating the Deep Core Muscles

Engaging Your Core for Stability and Strength

Overview:

The core muscles, including the transverse abdominis and pelvic floor muscles, are essential for stability and support in Pilates. In today's session, you'll learn how to activate these deep core muscles.

Activity:

1. Supine Pelvic Tilt: Knees bent and feet flat on the floor, lie on your back. Place your hands on your lower abdomen. Inhale to prepare, exhale, and gently tilt your pelvis up, pressing your lower back into the floor. Inhale to release. Repeat for 10 breath cycles.

2. **Pelvic Floor Engagement:** Sit comfortably on a chair or cushion. Imagine lifting the muscles of your pelvic floor as if you're trying to stop the flow of urine. Hold this engagement for a count of 5, then release. Repeat 10 times.

3. **Transverse Abdominis Activation:** Lie on your back with knees bent. Place your hands on your lower abdomen. Inhale deeply, and as you exhale, draw your navel toward your spine, engaging your transverse abdominis. Hold for 5 seconds, then release. Repeat for 10 cycles.

4. **Standing Core Engagement:** Stand with feet hip-width apart. Place your hands on your lower abdomen. Inhale deeply, and as you exhale, engage your deep core muscles, pulling your navel toward your spine. Hold for 5 seconds, then release. Repeat for 10 breath cycles.

5. **Core Awareness:** Throughout the day, practice engaging your deep core muscles during daily activities like sitting, walking, or even standing in line. This will help reinforce core awareness.

Day 4: Breathing Techniques for Mind-Body Connection

Breath Awareness and Coordination

Overview:

Breathing is integral to Pilates practice. It not only oxygenates your body but also enhances the mind-body connection. In today's session, you'll explore different breathing techniques to connect with your movements.

Activity:

1. Thoracic Breathing: Sit or stand comfortably. Place your hands on your ribcage, with your thumbs in the back and fingers in the front. Inhale deeply through your nose, expanding your ribcage to the sides and back. Exhale fully through your mouth, feeling your ribcage contract. Repeat for 10 breath cycles.

2. Diaphragmatic Breathing: Lie on your back with your knees bent and feet flat on the floor. Your chest and abdomen should be touched with one hand each. Deeply inhale through your nostrils while letting your chest remain still and allowing your abdomen to rise. Using your mouth to exhale, feel your belly drop.

3. Breath Coordination: Practice coordinating your breath with simple movements. For example, inhale as you reach your arms overhead, and exhale as you lower them. Focus on the smooth transition between breath and movement.

4. Mindful Breathing: Throughout the day, take moments to practice mindful breathing. Close your eyes, focus on your breath, and let go of any tension or stress with each exhale.

Day 5: Developing Pelvic Floor Strength

Building a Strong and Healthy Pelvic Floor

Overview:

A strong pelvic floor is essential for core stability, posture, and overall well-being. In today's session, you'll learn exercises to strengthen these crucial muscles.

Activity:

1. Pelvic Floor Lifts: Sit or lie down comfortably. Inhale deeply, and as you exhale, imagine lifting your pelvic floor muscles upward, as if you're trying to lift a small object. Inhale to release. Repeat for 10 breath cycles.

2. Elevator Exercise: Visualize your pelvic floor muscles like an elevator with four floors. With each exhale, lift the elevator to a different floor, gradually lifting higher with each breath cycle. Inhale to lower the elevator. Repeat for 10 cycles.

3. Bridge Pose with Pelvic Floor Engagement: Lie on your back with knees bent and feet flat on the floor. Inhale to prepare, exhale, and engage your pelvic floor muscles as you lift your hips off the floor into a bridge pose. Inhale to lower. Repeat for 10 repetitions.

4. Seated Activation: Sit on a chair or cushion. Inhale deeply, and as you exhale, lift your pelvic floor muscles. Hold for 5 seconds, then release. Repeat 10 times.

5. Daily Awareness: Throughout the day, remind yourself to engage your pelvic floor muscles during daily activities like standing up, walking, or bending over. This ongoing practice will help you maintain pelvic floor strength.

Day 6: Balance and Stability Exercises

Enhancing Balance and Coordination

Overview:

Balance and stability are essential for functional movement and injury prevention. In today's session, you'll engage in exercises that challenge your balance and enhance your stability.

Activity:

1. Single Leg Stance: Stand with your feet hip-width apart. Lift your right foot off the ground and shift your weight to your left leg. Select a focus for your attention and contract your core muscles to maintain stability. Switch legs after 30 seconds of holding.

2. Heel-to-Toe Walk: Take slow, deliberate steps by placing the heel of one foot directly in front of the toes of the other foot. This exercise challenges your balance and promotes proper alignment.

3. Tree Pose Variation: Stand on your left leg, bringing the sole of your right foot to your left calf or inner thigh. Find your balance, engage your core, and extend your arms overhead. Switch legs after 30 seconds of holding.

4. Wall Plank: Stand facing a wall, about an arm's length away. At shoulder height, place your palms against the wall. Lean forward and walk your feet back until your body forms a straight line from head to heels. Hold this position for 30 seconds, engaging your core for stability.

5. Weekly Progress Check: Reflect on your balance and stability improvements. Note any changes in your ability to maintain balance and how you feel physically during these exercises.

Day 7: Weekly Progress Check and Reflection

Reflecting on Your First Week

Overview:

Congratulations on completing your first week of the Pilates challenge! This day is dedicated to reflecting on your progress and setting intentions for the upcoming week.

Activity:

1. Progress Evaluation: Take a few moments to assess your progress. How do you feel after completing the activities of Week 1? Are you noticing changes in your posture, alignment, core engagement, or balance? Make notes in your journal or a dedicated space.

2. Weekly Goals: Set goals for the upcoming week. What specific aspects of your practice would you like to focus on? It could be deeper core engagement, improved alignment, or enhanced balance.

3. Positive Affirmations: Write down positive affirmations that you can repeat to yourself throughout the week. For instance, "I am laying a solid foundation for my Pilates journey" or "I am paying closer attention to the alignment of my body."

4. Mindfulness Practice: Spend a few minutes in quiet meditation or mindfulness. Focus on your breath and bring your awareness to the sensations in your body. This practice will help you cultivate a deeper mind-body connection.

Conclusion:

Week 1 of the 28 Days Wall Pilates Challenge for Women Over 50 has laid the groundwork for your journey. You've learned about posture, alignment, core engagement, breath coordination, pelvic floor strength, and balance. As you move into Week 2, carry these principles with you and continue to build upon the foundation you've established.

Remember, progress takes time, so be patient with yourself and celebrate each step forward in your Pilates practice.

CHAPTER 4

Week 2: Mobility and Flexibility Enhancement

Exploring Range of Motion and Flexibility

Goals for Week 2:

1. Enhance your spinal flexibility for improved posture.

2. Improve shoulder mobility and strength for functional movement.

3. Increase hip flexibility and range of motion for comfort and mobility.

4. Relieve tension in hamstrings and hip flexors for better flexibility.

5. Enhance joint mobility for overall movement health.

6. Embrace full-body flexibility through Pilates-inspired stretches.

Benefits for Week 2:

1. Improved Spinal Health: Enhance spinal flexibility to alleviate stiffness, reduce discomfort, and achieve better posture.

2. Functional Shoulder Movement: Increased shoulder mobility and strength enhance your ability to reach, lift, and perform daily tasks.

3. Enhanced Hip Comfort: Greater hip flexibility and range of motion contribute to comfortable movement and lower back health.

4. Reduced Muscle Tension: Release tension in hamstrings and hip flexors, improving flexibility and preventing discomfort.

5. Optimal Joint Function: Improved joint mobility supports fluid movement, reduces joint discomfort, and enhances overall range of motion.

6. Total Body Flexibility: Pilates-inspired stretches promote muscle relaxation, circulation, and a sense of overall well-being.

Welcome to Week 2 of the 28 Days Wall Pilates Challenge for Women Over 50. In this week, our focus shifts towards enhancing your mobility and flexibility. These qualities are crucial for maintaining joint health, preventing stiffness, and improving overall movement efficiency. We will guide you through each day's activities, offering detailed explanations to ensure you perform them correctly and safely.

Day 8: Increasing Spinal Flexibility

Exploring Spinal Mobility for Vitality

Overview:

Spinal flexibility is a key component of Pilates practice. A flexible spine contributes to better posture, reduced tension, and increased overall vitality. This session will introduce exercises designed to enhance the flexibility of your spine.

Activity:

1. Seated Spinal Rotation: Sit comfortably on the floor with your legs extended. Cross your right leg over your left, placing your right foot flat on the floor outside your left thigh. Inhale to prepare, exhale as you twist to the right, placing your left hand on your right knee and your right hand behind you for support. Inhale to lengthen your spine, exhale to deepen the twist. 30 seconds of holding, then switch sides.

2. Cat-Cow Stretch: Begin on your hands and knees in a tabletop position. Take a deep breath in as you lift your chin and tailbone in the cow stance. Exhale as you round your back, tucking your tailbone and chin to your chest (cat pose). Repeat this movement for 10 cycles, coordinating your breath.

3. Child's Pose with Rotation: From a kneeling position, sit back on your heels and extend your arms forward. Inhale to prepare, exhale, and reach your left arm under your right arm, rotating your torso to the right. Rest your left shoulder on the ground and hold for 30 seconds. Inhale to release, and switch sides.

4. Rolling Like a Ball: Sit on the floor, knees bent, feet flat. Hold onto your shins, round your spine, and lift your feet off the ground. Balance on your sit bones. Inhale as you roll back, exhale as you roll forward, balancing in a controlled manner. Repeat for 10 repetitions.

Day 9: Shoulder Mobility and Strength

Unlocking Shoulder Range of Motion

Overview:

Shoulder mobility is essential for many Pilates exercises and daily activities. This session focuses on improving the range of motion in your shoulders while also enhancing their strength and stability.

Activity:

1. Arm Circles: Stand tall with your arms extended at shoulder height. Start by creating little circles with your arms and progressively enlarge them. Reverse the direction after 10 circles. This exercise warms up your shoulder joints.

2. Shoulder Blade Squeezes: Sit or stand with your spine neutral. Imagine squeezing a pencil between your shoulder blades as you draw them together. Hold for five counts, then let go. Repeat for 10 repetitions.

3. Wall Angels: Stand with your back against a wall, feet a few inches away. Lift your arms, bringing your elbows and wrists to touch the wall. Slide your arms slowly up while keeping them in contact with the wall. Return to the starting position. Perform 10 reps.

4. Thread the Needle: Start on your hands and knees. Reach your right arm under your left arm, bringing your right shoulder and right cheek to the floor. Hold for 30 seconds, feeling the stretch in your upper back and shoulder. Inhale to release, and switch sides.

Day 10: Hip Flexibility and Range of Motion

Enhancing Hip Mobility for Better Movement

Overview:

Hip flexibility is vital for maintaining comfortable movement and preventing lower back discomfort. This session introduces exercises that target hip mobility, helping you move with greater ease.

Activity:

1. Hip Circles: Stand with your feet hip-width apart. Place your hands on your hips. Initiate circles by moving your hips in a circular motion. Perform 10 circles in one direction, then reverse. Your hip joints will warm up from this activity.

2. Hip Flexor Stretch: Lunging forward, take a step with your right foot. Drop your left knee to the ground. Push your hips forward slightly until you feel a stretch in the front of your left hip. 30 seconds of holding, then switch sides.

3. Pigeon Pose: Put your right knee behind your right wrist by bringing it forward. Keeping your hips square, extend your left leg behind you. Your forehead should be on the ground or a cushion as you lean forward. 30 seconds of holding, then switch sides.

4. Standing Hip Opener: Stand on your right leg, lifting your left knee to hip level. Hold onto your left ankle with your left hand, gently pulling your heel toward your left glute. Hold for 30 seconds, feeling the stretch in the front of your left thigh. Switch sides.

Day 11: Unlocking Hamstring and Hip Flexor Tightness

Relieving Tension in Hamstrings and Hip Flexors

Overview:

Tight hamstrings and hip flexors can contribute to discomfort and limited range of motion. This session targets these muscle groups, helping you release tension and improve flexibility.

Activity:

1. Hamstring Stretch: Sit on the floor with your legs extended. Hinge forward from your hips, reaching your hands toward your feet. According on your level of flexibility, hold onto your shins, ankles, or feet. Hold for 30 seconds, feeling the stretch in the back of your thighs.

2. Dynamic Hamstring Stretch: Stand with your feet hip-width apart. Step your right foot forward and flex your right foot. Hinge forward from your hips, reaching your hands toward your right foot. Keep your spine long and neutral. Return to the starting position after three counts of holding. Perform 10 repetitions on each side.

3. Hip Flexor Stretch: Kneel on your left knee and extend your right leg forward. Keep your hips square and press your pelvis forward slightly to feel a stretch in the front of your left hip. Hold for 30 seconds, then switch sides.

4. Dynamic Hip Flexor Stretch: Stand tall. Lunging forward, take a step back with your right foot. Bend your left knee and lower your hips, feeling a stretch in the front of your right hip. Push your hips forward slightly, then straighten your left leg to return to the starting position. Perform 10 repetitions on each side.

Day 12: Enhancing Joint Mobility Safely

Improving Joint Health and Mobility

Overview:

Maintaining healthy joints is crucial for overall mobility and longevity. This session incorporates exercises that promote joint health while also enhancing your flexibility.

Activity:

1. Ankle Circles: With your legs outstretched, sit down on the floor. Lift your right foot off the ground and make circles with your ankle. Perform 10 circles in each direction, then switch sides.

2. Wrist Mobility: Extend your right arm forward with your palm facing down. Use your left hand to gently press your right palm toward your forearm, creating a stretch in your wrist flexors. Switch sides after 20 seconds of holding.

3. Neck Mobility: Sit tall with your shoulders relaxed. Gently tilt your head to the right, bringing your right ear toward your right shoulder. Feel the stretch on your neck's left side while you hold the position for 15 seconds. Switch sides after returning to the center.

4. Shoulder Rolls: Stand or sit with your spine neutral. Roll your shoulders back and forth in a circular motion after raising them up toward your ears. 10 circles in each direction should be made.

Day 13: Pilates Stretches for Whole-Body Flexibility

Comprehensive Stretching for Total Flexibility

Overview:

Today's session combines Pilates-inspired stretches to enhance flexibility throughout your entire body. These stretches are designed to lengthen your muscles, improve circulation, and promote relaxation.

Activity:

1. Chest Opener: Place your feet hip-width apart as you stand. When lifting your arms away from your body, gently interlace your fingers behind your back. Feel the stretch in your chest and shoulders. Hold for 30 seconds.

2. Seated Forward Fold: Sit on the floor with your legs extended. Inhale to lengthen your spine, then exhale as you hinge forward from your hips, reaching your hands toward your feet. According on your level of flexibility, hold onto your shins, ankles, or feet. Hold for 30 seconds.

3. Spinal Twist: Sit on the floor with your legs extended. Bend your right knee and place your right foot on the outside of your left knee. Inhale to lengthen your spine, then exhale as you twist to the right, placing your left elbow on the outside of your right knee. 30 seconds of holding, then switch sides.

4. Standing Forward Fold: Stand with your feet hip-width apart. Inhale to lengthen your spine, then exhale as you hinge forward from your hips. Let your upper body hang down, reaching for your shins, ankles, or the floor. Hold for 30 seconds.

5. Total Body Stretch: Lie on your back with your arms extended overhead and your legs straight. Inhale deeply, then exhale as you simultaneously reach your arms overhead and point your toes away from your body. Feel the stretch throughout your entire body. Hold for 20 seconds.

Day 14: Weekly Progress Check and Reflection

Reflecting on Your Second Week

Overview:

Congratulations on completing the second week of the Pilates challenge! It's time to reflect on your progress and set intentions for the upcoming week focused on strength and muscle tone development.

Activity:

1. Progress Evaluation: Take a moment to assess your progress in terms of mobility and flexibility. Are you noticing increased range of motion, reduced tension, or improved joint comfort? Make notes in your journal or a dedicated space.

2. Weekly Goals: Set goals for the next week. What specific aspects of your mobility and flexibility would you like to focus on? Whether it's deepening a stretch or improving joint mobility, outline your intentions.

3. Positive Affirmations: Write down positive affirmations related to your flexibility journey. For instance, "I am honoring my body's need for flexibility" or "I am cultivating a flexible and mobile body."

4. Mindfulness Practice: Dedicate a few minutes to a mindfulness practice. Pay attention to your breathing and your body's sensations. Embrace the feeling of increased flexibility and mobility as you move forward in your Pilates journey.

Conclusion:

You've explored spinal flexibility, shoulder mobility, hip range of motion, joint health, and full-body stretches. mobility and flexibility.

CHAPTER 5

Week 3: Strength and Muscle Tone Development

Empowering Your Muscles with Strength Training

Goals for week 3:

1. Understand the fundamentals of resistance training.

2. Build upper body strength and muscle tone.

3. Strengthen your lower body muscles for improved stability.

4. Integrate core engagement into strength exercises.

5. Perform full-body resistance exercises for comprehensive strength.

6. Incorporate small equipment to intensify your strength training.

Benefits for week 3:

1. Upper Body Strength: Build strength in your upper body, including shoulders, chest, back, and arms, enhancing functional abilities.

2. Lower Body Stability: Strengthen lower body muscles to improve balance, stability, and overall coordination.

3. Core Stability: Integrate core engagement into strength exercises for improved posture, balance, and spinal support.

4. Comprehensive Strength: Perform full-body resistance exercises that target multiple muscle groups for enhanced overall strength.

5. Intensified Training: Incorporate small equipment to intensify your workouts, adding resistance for greater muscle activation.

6. Increased Confidence: Developing strength and muscle tone boosts your self-confidence and enhances your physical capabilities.

Welcome to Week 3 of the 28 Days Wall Pilates Challenge for Women Over 50. This week, we dive into the realm of strength and muscle tone development. Strengthening your muscles not only enhances your physical capabilities but also contributes to improved posture, stability, and overall vitality. Join us as we guide you through each day's activities, offering detailed instructions to ensure your success.

Day 15: Introduction to Pilates Resistance Training

Discovering the Power of Resistance Training

Overview:

Welcome to Week 3, where we introduce resistance training to build strength and muscle tone. Resistance exercises challenge your muscles by adding external resistance, such as bands or weights. Today, we'll focus on the foundational concepts of resistance training.

Activity:

1. Understanding Resistance: Learn about the different types of resistance, including body weight, resistance bands, and dumbbells. Understand how resistance training targets specific muscle groups to build strength.

2. Selecting Appropriate Resistance: If using resistance bands, choose a band with appropriate tension for your fitness level. If using dumbbells, start with light weights and gradually increase as needed.

3. Importance of Proper Form: Emphasize the importance of maintaining proper form throughout each exercise. Proper form ensures effectiveness and reduces the risk of injury.

Day 16: Building Upper Body Strength

Empowering Your Upper Body Muscles

Overview:

Today's session focuses on building strength in your upper body, including the shoulders, chest, back, and arms. These exercises will enhance your upper body muscle tone and functional strength.

Activity:

1. Resistance Band Rows: Attach a resistance band to a secure anchor point. Hold the band handles in each hand. Step back to create tension. Pull the bands toward your torso, squeezing your shoulder blades together. Slowly release. Perform 3 sets of 12 reps.

2. Push-Ups: Perform modified push-ups (on knees) or standard push-ups. Engage your core and maintain a straight line with your body. Perform 3 sets of 10 reps.

3. Dumbbell Shoulder Press: Sit or stand with a dumbbell in each hand at shoulder height. As you press the dumbbells overhead, extend your arms fully. Slowly lower. Perform 3 sets of 10 reps.

4. Resistance Band Bicep Curls: Stand on a resistance band, holding the handles. Contract your biceps as you curl the bands toward your shoulders. Slowly release. Perform 3 sets of 12 reps.

Day 17: Lower Body Muscle Activation

Engaging and Strengthening Lower Body Muscles

Overview:

Today's exercises focus on activating and strengthening the muscles of your lower body, including the glutes, quadriceps, hamstrings, and calves. Building lower body strength contributes to better posture and overall stability.

Activity:

1. Resistance Band Squats: Place a resistance band above your knees. Stand with feet hip-width apart. Perform squats, pressing your knees against the resistance of the band. Perform 3 sets of 12 reps.

2. Lunges: Step forward with your right foot, lowering your left knee toward the ground. In order to get back to the beginning position, push through your right heel. Legs are alternated. On each leg, complete 3 sets of 10 repetitions.

3. Dumbbell Deadlifts: Hold a dumbbell in each hand in front of your thighs. Hinge at your hips, lowering the dumbbells toward the ground while keeping your back straight. Return to the starting position. Perform 3 sets of 10 reps.

4. Calf Raises: Place your feet hip-width apart as you stand. Lift your heels as high as you can, balancing on the balls of your feet. Lower your heels back down. Perform 3 sets of 15 reps.

Day 18: Core Strengthening Progressions

Advancing Your Core Strength

Overview:

Building on your core awareness from Week 1, today's session introduces more advanced core exercises to enhance strength and stability. A strong core supports better posture and helps prevent injuries.

Activity:

1. Plank Variations: Start with forearm plank or full plank. Engage your core and keep your body in a straight line from head to heels. Hold for 30 to 60 seconds.

2. Leg Raises: Lie on your back with your legs extended. Keep your legs straight as you raise them off the ground. Slowly lower them without touching the ground. Perform 3 sets of 12 reps.

3. Bicycle Crunches: With your hands behind your head, lie on your back. As you stretch your right leg, bring your right elbow near your left knee. Alternate sides in a cycling motion. Perform 3 sets of 20 reps.

4. Side Plank: Lie on your right side, supporting your body on your right forearm. As you form a straight line from your head to your feet, raise your hips off the ground. Hold for 30 seconds, then switch sides.

Day 19: Full-Body Resistance Exercises

Integrating Strength into Full-Body Movements

Overview:

Today's session combines various resistance exercises to engage multiple muscle groups simultaneously, providing a comprehensive full-body workout.

Activity:

1. Squat to Shoulder Press: Hold a dumbbell in each hand at shoulder height. Perform a squat, then press the dumbbells overhead as you stand. Return to the starting position. Perform 3 sets of 10 reps.

2. Push-Up to Renegade Row: Perform a push-up, then lift one dumbbell to your hip while balancing on the opposite hand. Alternate sides with each push-up. Perform 3 sets of 10 reps.

3. Squat Thrusters: Hold a dumbbell in each hand at shoulder height. Perform a squat, then explosively stand up, pressing the dumbbells overhead. Perform 3 sets of 10 reps.

4. Burpees: Begin in a standing position. Drop into a squat, place your hands on the ground, jump your feet back to a plank position, perform a push-up, jump your feet back to the squat position, and explosively jump up. Perform 3 sets of 8 reps.

Day 20: Incorporating Small Equipment for Added Challenge

Utilizing Small Equipment for Increased Resistance

Overview:

Incorporating small equipment, such as resistance bands and small weights, can intensify your strength training. This session introduces exercises that leverage small equipment for added challenge.

Activity:

1. Resistance Band Leg Press: Attach a resistance band to a secure anchor point. Place the band around your ankles. Stand with feet hip-width apart. Step back to create tension. Perform squats, pressing your knees against the resistance of the band. Perform 3 sets of 12 reps.

2. Dumbbell Rows with Bands: Secure a resistance band to a wall or anchor point. Hold a dumbbell in each hand. Step back to create tension in the band. Perform rows, squeezing your shoulder blades together. Perform 3 sets of 12 reps.

3. Banded Glute Bridges: Place a resistance band above your knees. Knees bent and feet flat, lie on your back. Using your glutes, raise your hips off the ground. Perform 3 sets of 15 reps.

4. Resistance Band Triceps Extensions: Attach a resistance band to a secure anchor point. Hold the band handle in one hand. Extend your arm overhead, then bend your elbow to perform triceps extensions. Perform 3 sets of 12 reps on each arm.

Day 21: Weekly Progress Check and Reflection

Reflecting on Your Third Week

Overview:

Congratulations on completing the third week of the Pilates challenge focused on strength and muscle tone development. This is an opportune time to reflect on your progress and set intentions for the final week.

Activity:

1. Progress Evaluation: Assess your progress in terms of strength gains and muscle tone improvements. Have you noticed increased muscle definition, enhanced strength, or improved functional abilities? Document your observations.

2. Weekly Goals: Set goals for the final week of the challenge. Consider what specific areas of strength and muscle development you want to focus on, whether it's increasing resistance or fine-tuning form.

3. Positive Affirmations: Write down positive affirmations related to your strength journey. Examples are "I am gaining strength with every workout" and "Strength training has given me more confidence."

4. Mindfulness Practice: Spend a few moments in mindful reflection. Focus on the sensations in your body, acknowledging the changes you've experienced during the strength-focused week.

Conclusion:

As you conclude Week 3 of the 28 Days Wall Pilates Challenge for Women Over 50, celebrate your dedication to building strength and enhancing muscle tone. You've explored resistance training, upper body and lower body exercises, core strengthening, and the use of small equipment. The strength you've gained over these three weeks will empower you in your daily activities and contribute to your overall well-being. As you transition into the final week, which focuses on balance and coordination, remember that strength is a journey, and every effort you invest brings you closer to your goals.

CHAPTER 6

Week 4: Balance and Coordination Enhancement

Mastering Balance and Coordination Skills

Goals for week 4:

1. Recognize the importance of balance and coordination in daily life.

2. Develop a foundation for balance through basic exercises.

3. Integrate core engagement into advanced balance exercises.

4. Challenge your balance and coordination with dynamic movements.

5. Fuse balance challenges with strength elements for stability.

6. Create a seamless flow of balanced movements for coordination.

Benefits for week 4:

1. Enhanced Stability: Develop balance through targeted exercises, reducing the risk of falls and improving overall stability.

2. Improved Coordination: Practice coordinated movements that enhance your ability to perform tasks with fluidity and precision.

3. Core Strength Integration: Strengthen your core muscles while challenging your balance, improving stability and posture.

4. Functional Movement: Dynamic balance exercises improve your ability to navigate daily activities and movement challenges.

5. Full-Body Harmony: Combining balance challenges with strength elements fosters harmonious movement and coordination.

6. Mind-Body Connection: Improved balance and coordination deepen your mind-body connection, enhancing body awareness.

Welcome to the final week of the 28 Days Wall Pilates Challenge for Women Over 50. In Week 4, our focus shifts to enhancing your balance and coordination. These skills are integral to functional movement, posture, and injury prevention. We'll guide you through each day's activities, providing detailed explanations to ensure you perform them effectively and safely.

Day 22: Understanding Balance and Coordination

Exploring the Importance of Balance and Coordination

Overview:

Welcome to Week 4, where we delve into the realm of balance and coordination. These skills are vital for maintaining stability, preventing falls, and executing movements with precision. Today, we'll explore the importance of balance and coordination in daily life and Pilates practice.

Activity:

1. Balancing Act: Reflect on how balance impacts your everyday activities, from walking to reaching for items on a shelf. Consider how improved balance can enhance your quality of life.

2. Coordination Connection: Recognize the connection between coordination and efficient movement. Coordination involves the harmonious interaction of different muscle groups to perform tasks smoothly.

Day 23: Basic Balance Exercises

Building a Foundation for Balance

Overview:

Today's session introduces basic balance exercises to lay the foundation for enhanced stability. These exercises focus on engaging core muscles and developing proprioception.

Activity:

1. Single Leg Stand: Stand on your left leg, lifting your right foot off the ground. Focus on a stationary point to help maintain balance. Switch legs after 30 seconds of holding. Attempt three sets on each leg.

2. Tightrope Walk: Imagine a tightrope on the ground. Walking with one foot in front of the other along the fictitious line. Engage your core for stability. Walk for 20 steps.

3. Heel-to-Toe Balance: Stand with your right heel against your left toes. Focus on maintaining your balance as you walk forward, placing your left heel against your right toes with each step. Walk for 20 steps.

Day 24: Advanced Balance and Core Integration

Integrating Core Engagement into Balance

Overview:

Today's session combines balance exercises with core engagement. This integration enhances your ability to stabilize your body while executing coordinated movements.

Activity:

1. Tree Pose: Stand on your left leg. Put your right foot's sole against the calf or inner thigh of your left leg. Extend your arms overhead. Engage your core for balance. Switch legs after 30 seconds of holding.

2. Warrior III Pose: Stand on your left leg, extending your right leg behind you. Lean forward as you extend your arms forward. Keep your hips square and engage your core for balance. Hold for 30 seconds, then switch legs.

3. Modified Plank Leg Lift: Begin in a modified plank position (on your knees). Straighten your right leg as you raise it off the ground. To keep yourself stable, contract your core. Each leg should be lifted for three sets of ten.

Day 25: Dynamic Balance and Coordination Challenges

Enhancing Balance Through Movement

Overview:

Dynamic balance exercises challenge your stability while incorporating movement. Today's session introduces exercises that require coordination and control as you move.

Activity:

1. Lateral Leg Lifts: Stand on your left leg. Straightening your right leg, extend it to the side. Engage your core for balance. Lower your leg and repeat for 10 reps. Switch legs and repeat.

2. Cross-Body Toe Touches: Stand on your left leg. Reach your right hand toward your left foot, crossing your body. Repeat on the other side, then go back to your starting position. On each side, complete 3 sets of 10 repetitions.

3. Balancing Bird: Stand on your left leg, extending your right leg straight behind you. Reach your right arm forward and extend your left arm back. Obtain and maintain balance for 20 seconds. Switch sides and repeat.

Day 26: Integrating Balance and Strength

Fusing Balance and Strength Elements

Overview:

Today's exercises combine balance challenges with strength elements. This fusion enhances your ability to stabilize your body while engaging various muscle groups.

Activity:

1. Single Leg Squats: Stand on your left leg. Bend your left knee and lower your body into a squat, extending your right leg straight in front of you. In order to get back to the beginning position, push through your left heel. On each leg, complete 3 sets of 10 repetitions.

2. Warrior II Pose with Arm Lift: Stand with your legs wide apart. Turn your right foot out and bend your right knee. Extend your arms to the sides, parallel to the ground. Lift your left leg off the ground and extend your left arm overhead. Switch sides after 20 seconds of holding.

3. Balance Ball Taps: Stand on your left leg. Hold a small ball in your hands. Tap the ball to the ground on your right side, then lift it overhead on your left side. Perform 3 sets of 10 taps on each side.

Day 27: Balance and Coordination Flow

Seamless Flow of Balanced Movements

Overview:

Today's session involves a flow of balanced movements, combining exercises to create a harmonious sequence that challenges your stability and coordination.

Activity:

1. Flow Sequence: Begin with a single leg stand on your left leg. Transition into a tree pose on your left leg. From there, move into a modified plank leg lift with your left knee lifted. Complete the flow on your left side, then repeat on your right side.

Day 28: Final Progress Check and Reflection

Celebrating Your Journey

Overview:

Congratulations on reaching the final day of the Pilates challenge! This day is dedicated to reflecting on your progress, celebrating your achievements, and setting intentions for your continued wellness journey.

Activity:

1. Progress Evaluation: Take time to reflect on your journey through the challenge. How have you improved in terms of balance, coordination, strength, and overall well-being? Celebrate your accomplishments.

2. Weekly Goals: Set intentions for your ongoing wellness journey. Consider how you will incorporate the lessons and practices from the challenge into your daily life.

3. Positive Affirmations: Write down positive affirmations that inspire you to maintain your balance, coordination, and overall health. For instance, "I am capable of moving with grace and stability" or "I am embracing my body's innate balance."

4. Mindfulness Practice: Dedicate a few minutes to mindful reflection. Focus on the sensations in your body and the sense of accomplishment you've achieved during the four-week journey.

Conclusion:

Congratulations on completing the "28 Days Wall Pilates Challenge for Women Over 50." Throughout this transformative journey, you've explored posture, alignment, core engagement, breath coordination, pelvic floor strength, flexibility, strength, balance, and coordination. Your commitment to your well-being is commendable, and the skills you've cultivated will continue to support you in your daily life. As you move beyond this challenge, remember that wellness is an ongoing pursuit. Embrace the balance, strength, and coordination you've gained, and carry them forward to create a vibrant and empowered life.

Conclusion

Celebrating Your Pilates Journey

Congratulations on completing the 28 Days Wall Pilates Challenge for Women Over 50! As you conclude this transformative journey, take a moment to celebrate your achievements and reflect on the profound changes you've experienced, both physically and mentally. This concluding chapter serves as a reflection on the significance of your Pilates journey and offers guidance on how to carry the benefits forward in your daily life.

Reflecting on Your Journey:

Take a moment to look back on the past four weeks. Consider the progress you've made in terms of strength, flexibility, and balance. Reflect on the mindfulness and self-awareness you've cultivated through daily practice. Acknowledge any physical or mental shifts you've experienced during this challenge.

The Mind-Body Connection:

Throughout the challenge, you've explored the powerful connection between your mind and body. Pilates is not just a physical exercise but a practice that encourages holistic well-being. As you conclude this journey, remember the importance of this mind-body synergy. Carry the mindfulness and intentionality you've embraced during Pilates into other aspects of your life, promoting a sense of balance and clarity.

Maintaining a Consistent Practice:

While the challenge has officially concluded, Pilates can continue to be an integral part of your daily routine. Consider integrating Pilates into your ongoing fitness regimen. Whether you practice for a few minutes each day or engage in longer sessions a few times a week, maintaining consistency is key to preserving the benefits you've gained.

Setting New Goals:

As you move forward, consider setting new goals for your Pilates practice. Perhaps you wish to explore more advanced exercises, deepen your flexibility, or focus on specific muscle groups. Setting clear goals keeps your practice dynamic and motivating, providing a sense of purpose.

Incorporating Mindfulness:

The mindfulness you've cultivated during this challenge can extend beyond your Pilates practice. Embrace moments of mindfulness in your daily life. Whether it's through conscious breathing, mindful movement, or simply being present in the moment, this practice can reduce stress and enhance your overall well-being.

Connecting with a Community:

Consider joining a local or online Pilates community to connect with like-minded individuals. Sharing your experiences, challenges, and successes with others can provide a sense of camaraderie and motivation on your fitness journey.

Maintaining Safety and Self-Care:

Above all, prioritize safety and self-care. Continue to heed the safety tips and precautions you've learned during the challenge. Listen to your body, adjust exercises as needed, and seek professional guidance if you have any specific health concerns.

Your Pilates Journey Continues:

Remember that your Pilates journey is an ongoing process. It's not about reaching a destination but about embracing the journey itself. The physical and mental benefits of Pilates are long-lasting and can positively impact various aspects of your life.

As you conclude this 28 Days Wall Pilates Challenge, celebrate your dedication and commitment to your well-being. Know that the journey you've embarked upon is not finite but rather a continuous exploration of self-improvement, strength, and mindfulness. Carry the lessons and benefits of Pilates with you as you navigate the path ahead, and may your newfound vitality and balance serve as a source of inspiration for the days, weeks, and years to come.

28-day challenge

Today's activity:

Why is this important for me:

Strenghts:

Weaknesses:

benefits:

days

How did it go:

What did I learn:

28-day challenge

Today's activity: _____

Why is this important for me: _____

_____

Strenghts: _____

Weaknesses: _____

benefits: _____

days

→ ◯—◯—◯—◯—◯—◯—◯—◯—◯

◯—◯—◯—◯—◯—◯—◯—◯—◯

◯—◯—◯—◯—◯—◯—◯

How did it go: _____

_____

What did I learn: _____

_____

28-day challenge

Today's activity: _____

Why is this important for me: _____

_____

Strenghts: _____

Weaknesses: _____

benefits: _____

_____

days

How did it go: _____

_____

What did I learn: _____

_____

_____

28-day challenge

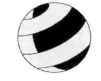

Today's activity: _____

Why is this important for me: _____

_____

Strenghts: _____

Weaknesses: _____

benefits: _____

days

⇒ ◯—◯—◯—◯ ◯—◯—◯—◯—◯

◯—◯—◯—◯—◯—◯—◯—◯—◯—◯

◯—◯—◯—◯—◯—◯—◯—◯___

How did it go: _____

_____

What did I learn: _____

_____

_____

28-day challenge

Today's activity: _____

Why is this important for me: _____
_____

Strenghts: _____

Weaknesses: _____

benefits: _____
_____

days

How did it go: _____
_____

What did I learn: _____
_____
_____

28-day challenge

Today's activity: _____

Why is this important for me: _____

_____

Strenghts: _____

Weaknesses: _____

benefits: _____

days

How did it go: _____

_____

What did I learn: _____

_____

28-day challenge

Today's activity: _____

Why is this important for me: _____

_____

Strenghts: _____

Weaknesses: _____

benefits: _____

days

How did it go: _____

_____

What did I learn: _____

_____

_____

28-day challenge

Today's activity: _____

Why is this important for me: _____

_____

Strenghts: _____

Weaknesses: _____

benefits: _____

days

⟹ ◯—◯—◯—◯—◯—◯—◯—◯—◯

◯—◯—◯—◯—◯—◯—◯—◯—◯

◯—◯—◯—◯—◯—◯—◯—◯——

How did it go: _____

_____

What did I learn: _____

_____

28-day challenge

Today's activity: _____

Why is this important for me: _____

_____

Strenghts: _____

Weaknesses: _____

benefits: _____

days

How did it go: _____

_____

What did I learn: _____

_____

28-day challenge

Today's activity: _____

Why is this important for me: _____

_____

Strenghts: _____

Weaknesses: _____

benefits: _____

days

→ ◯ ◯ ◯ ◯ ◯ ◯ ◯ ◯ ◯

◯ ◯ ◯ ◯ ◯ ◯ ◯ ◯ ◯

◯ ◯ ◯ ◯ ◯ ◯ ◯

How did it go: _____

_____

What did I learn: _____

_____

28-day challenge

Today's activity: _____

Why is this important for me: _____

_____

Strenghts: _____

Weaknesses: _____

benefits: _____

_____

days

How did it go: _____

_____

What did I learn: _____

_____

_____

28-day challenge

Today's activity: _____

Why is this important for me: _____
_____

Strenghts: _____

Weaknesses: _____

benefits: _____
_____

days

⇨ ◯—◯—◯—◯ ◯—◯—◯—◯—◯

◯—◯—◯—◯—◯—◯—◯—◯—◯

◯—◯—◯—◯—◯—◯—◯—◯

How did it go: _____
_____

What did I learn: _____
_____

28-day challenge

Today's activity: _____

Why is this important for me: _____

_____

Strenghts: _____

Weaknesses: _____

benefits: _____

days

How did it go: _____

_____

What did I learn: _____

_____

_____

28-day challenge

Today's activity: _____

Why is this important for me: _____

_____

Strenghts: _____

Weaknesses: _____

benefits: _____

days

⇨ ○─○─○─○─○─○─○─○─○

○─○─○─○─○─○─○─○─○

○─○─○─○─○─○─○

How did it go: _____

_____

What did I learn: _____

_____

28-day challenge

Today's activity: _____

Why is this important for me: _____

_____

Strenghts: _____

Weaknesses: _____

benefits: _____

days

⇨ ◯—◯—◯—◯—◯—◯—◯—◯—◯
◯—◯—◯—◯—◯—◯—◯—◯—◯
◯—◯—◯—◯—◯—◯—◯

How did it go: _____

_____

What did I learn: _____

_____

_____

28-day challenge

Today's activity: _____

Why is this important for me: _____

_____

Strenghts: _____

Weaknesses: _____

benefits: _____

days

→ ◯—◯—◯—◯ ◯—◯—◯—◯—◯

◯—◯—◯—◯ ◯—◯—◯—◯—◯

◯—◯—◯—◯ ◯—◯—◯—◯

How did it go: _____

_____

What did I learn: _____

_____

28-day challenge

Today's activity: _____

Why is this important for me: _____

_____

Strenghts: _____

Weaknesses: _____

benefits: _____

_____

days

→ ◯—◯—◯—◯—◯—◯—◯—◯—◯

◯—◯—◯—◯—◯—◯—◯—◯—◯

◯—◯—◯—◯—◯—◯—◯—◯

How did it go: _____

_____

What did I learn: _____

_____

_____

28-day challenge

Today's activity: _____

Why is this important for me: _____

_____

Strenghts: _____

Weaknesses: _____

benefits: _____

days

How did it go: _____

_____

What did I learn: _____

_____

28-day challenge

Today's activity: _____

Why is this important for me: _____

_____

Strenghts: _____

Weaknesses: _____

benefits: _____

days

⇨ ◯—◯—◯—◯—◯—◯—◯—◯—◯

◯—◯—◯—◯—◯—◯—◯—◯—◯

◯—◯—◯—◯—◯—◯—◯—◯

How did it go: _____

_____

What did I learn: _____

_____

_____

28-day challenge

Today's activity: _____

Why is this important for me: _____

_____

Strenghts: _____

Weaknesses: _____

benefits: _____

days

⟹ ◯—◯—◯—◯ ◯—◯—◯—◯—◯

◯—◯—◯—◯ ◯—◯—◯—◯—◯

◯—◯—◯—◯ ◯—◯—◯—◯

How did it go: _____

_____

What did I learn: _____

_____

96

28-day challenge

Today's activity: _____

Why is this important for me: _____

_____

Strenghts: _____

Weaknesses: _____

benefits: _____

days

⇨ ◯—◯—◯—◯—◯—◯—◯—◯—◯

◯—◯—◯—◯—◯—◯—◯—◯—◯

◯—◯—◯—◯—◯—◯—◯

How did it go: _____

_____

What did I learn: _____

_____

28-day challenge

Today's activity: _____

Why is this important for me: _____

_____

Strenghts: _____

Weaknesses: _____

benefits: _____

days

How did it go: _____

_____

What did I learn: _____

_____

28-day challenge

Today's activity: _____

Why is this important for me: _____

_____

Strenghts: _____

Weaknesses: _____

benefits: _____

days

⟹ ◯—◯—◯—◯—◯—◯—◯—◯

◯—◯—◯—◯—◯—◯—◯—◯—◯

◯—◯—◯—◯—◯—◯—◯—

How did it go: _____

_____

What did I learn: _____

_____

_____

28-day challenge

Today's activity: _____

Why is this important for me: _____

_____

Strenghts: _____

Weaknesses: _____

benefits: _____

days

How did it go: _____

_____

What did I learn: _____

_____

28-day challenge

Today's activity: _____

Why is this important for me: _____
_____

Strenghts: _____

Weaknesses: _____

benefits: _____

days

How did it go: _____
_____

What did I learn: _____
_____

28-day challenge

Today's activity: _____

Why is this important for me: _____

_____

Strenghts: _____

Weaknesses: _____

benefits: _____

days

How did it go: _____

_____

What did I learn: _____

_____

_____

28-day challenge

Today's activity: _____

Why is this important for me: _____

_____

Strenghts: _____

Weaknesses: _____

benefits: _____

days

How did it go: _____

_____

What did I learn: _____

_____

28-day challenge

Today's activity: _____

Why is this important for me: _____

_____

Strenghts: _____

Weaknesses: _____

benefits: _____

days

→ ◯—◯—◯—◯—◯—◯—◯—◯—◯

◯—◯—◯—◯—◯—◯—◯—◯—◯

◯—◯—◯—◯—◯—◯—◯————

How did it go: _____

_____

What did I learn: _____

_____

Made in the USA
Columbia, SC
25 November 2024

47594609R00059